INTERNATIONAL SURVEY OF MEDICAL & OTHER LIFE SCIENCES FACULTY: EVALUATION OF THE LIBRARY

ISBN 978-1-57440-456-2

Table of Contents

SUMMARY OF MAIN FINDINGS

What Patrons Like Most About their Medical and Other Life Sciences Libraries

We started the survey by asking a simple open-ended question: What do you most like about the scientific and scholarly resources of your academic or medical library? Overwhelmingly, the depth and quality of online resources was the most significant factor cited, followed by the helpfulness of the library staff. Good quality interlibrary loan was also mentioned by multiple participants as well as the broad range of journal subscriptions, in whatever format.

What Patrons Like Least About their Medical and Other Life Sciences Libraries

In general, limitations on journal availability is the primary complaint. The physical distance of library resources from laboratories was another common complaint.

Frequency of Visiting the Medical or Life Sciences Library

The scholars sampled visited their academic or medical library a mean of 2.22 times in the past 30 days with a range of 0 to 50 times. The more highly ranked the university, the fewer actual library visitors did the library receive. Those ranked in the top 25 worldwide received a mean of 1.52 while those ranked lower than 135 received a mean of 3.76 visits per survey participant. Lecturers and instructors were the most frequent visitors, professors the leas frequent; the former visited a mean of 7 times in the past 30 days, the latter, only 0.48 times.

Level of Satisfaction with Medical or Life Sciences Interlibrary Loan Services

We asked: how satisfied are you with your academic library's inter-library loan services? We gave five answers to this multiple-choice question, which were: Highly Satisfied, Satisfied, Somewhat Satisfied, Dissatisfied and Highly Dissatisfied. Overall, 32.18% of those sampled did not answer the question, while a plurality of 35.63% said that they were satisfied and 24.24%, highly satisfied. Only 6.9% were only somewhat satisfied and 1.15% dissatisfied; none were highly dissatisfied.

Universities in the top 25 worldwide had the best satisfaction ratings in inter-library loan, with 34.1% highly satisfied vs. between 17.8% to 24.4% for the other cohorts. Also, universities charging the lowest annual tuition had far fewer who were highly satisfied, only 11.11% vs those in higher tuition ranges. It may be that universities with more modest funding may not be able to spend enough on interlibrary loan to be competitive with their better funded peers. Indeed, private universities significantly outperformed public ones in this arena, with more than twice the percentage of respondents (37.3%) indicating high satisfaction compared to public colleges (17.4%). Satisfaction tended to decline with the age of the survey respondent, excepting for the very youngest; 30.2% of those aged 31-39 were highly satisfied with interlibrary loan services vs only 17.86% of those aged 60 or over. Also, quite strikingly, faculty in medical schools are far more satisfied with interlibrary loan services than are faculty in biology or chemistry departments, or schools of public health or dental or veterinary schools. Indeed, only 6.45% of those in biology departments, and 7.69% of those in chemistry departments, were highly satisfied vs, 35.11% of those in medical school faculties of all kinds.

Level of Satisfaction with Medical or Life Sciences Library eBook Collection & Services

Satisfaction with eBook collections was somewhat less pronounced. 26.44% did not answer the question; a plurality of 39.08% were satisfied and 21.26% satisfied while 10.92% were somewhat satisfied and 2.3% dissatisfied; none were highly dissatisfied. In Australia/New Zealand 30% were only somewhat satisfied and this may reflect the generally more demanding attitude of library patrons in these countries since they tend to rely more on eBooks than is the case in other locales. It may be a question of service but it seems more likely a question of stronger relative need, and greater expectations.
Only 4.88% of faculty sampled in universities with a US News & World Report ranking below 135 were highly satisfied with their eBook collections, much lower satisfaction ratings than for more highly ranked universities. Satisfaction also correlated relatively strongly with tuition; in general, with exception, the higher the tuition charged the greater the satisfaction with the library eBook collection. Once again private colleges vastly outperformed public ones.

Untenured faculty were happier than tenured faculty, among whom only 11.36% were highly satisfied. Again, medical school faculty were much happier than others. Nearly 30% of medical school faculty were highly satisfied while only 3.7% of faculty in public health, nursing or health informatics felt the same.

Level of Satisfaction with Medical or Life Sciences Library Subject Specialists

Next we asked about how satisfied respondents were with the level of knowledge of the library's subject specialists. More than 39% did not answer the question while a plurality of 30.46% were satisfied but only 16.67% were highly satisfied and 11.49%, somewhat satisfied; 1.72% were dissatisfied and 0.57%, highly dissatisfied. Only 10% of faculty sampled from Australia/New Zealand were highly satisfied though 50% were satisfied. Once again, satisfaction was highly correlated with university ranking; the higher the ranking, the greater the level of satisfaction with the knowledge level of the university library subject specialist. For those in the top 24, 27.27% were highly satisfied, but this percentage drops to 20.45% for those tanked 25-90 and then to 11.11% for those in the91-135 cohort; it finally bottoms out at 7.32% for universities ranked below 135. Unlike in other areas, professors tended to be more satisfied than others; nearly 23% of them were highly satisfied with their subject librarian's knowledge level of their subject while only 3.85% of associate professors or readers had the same judgement. Differences between medical school and other life sciences faculty in this area were not pronounced.

Level of Satisfaction with Medical or Life Sciences Library Database Offerings in Your Field

We asked: how satisfied were survey participants with the access to databases in your field? Only 14.94% did not answer the question while a plurality of 37.36% were satisfied and 35.06% highly satisfied; 9.2% were only somewhat satisfied and 1.72% dissatisfied and the same percentage, highly dissatisfied. Satisfaction was greatest overall in Australia/New Zealand where 90% were highly satisfied or satisfied. Private universities and universities at higher tuition levels tended to have higher levels of satisfaction than their counterparts but the differences were not as great as for some other library services.

Level of Satisfaction with Medical or Life Sciences Library's Journal Collection

Next, we asked about the level of satisfaction with the breadth and quality of the library's journal collection; only 12.64% did not answer the question. A plurality of 35.06% were satisfied and 34.48% highly satisfied while 10.92% were somewhat satisfied and 6.32% dissatisfied; 0.57% were highly dissatisfied. Satisfaction was highest in the USA where 40.15% were highly satisfied vs. only 12% in the UK/Ireland. Once again satisfaction was highly correlated with university ranking; for those in the top 24, 50% were highly satisfied while only 9.76% of those in the lowest quartile in the sample, below a world rank of 135, were highly satisfied.

Level of Satisfaction with Medical or Life Sciences Data Archiving and Data Curation Services

We asked about satisfaction levels with the library's data archiving and data curation services.

42.53% did not answer the question; 20.11% were highly satisfied and 24.71% satisfied while 9.77% were only somewhat satisfied and 2.3%, dissatisfied; 0.57% were highly dissatisfied. High levels of satisfaction were most common in the USA and in the more highly ranked universities. In the universities ranked below 135 only 9.76% were highly satisfied with the data management and curation services of the library. Overwhelmingly, younger scholars were happier than older ones with data archiving and curation services. For those under age 40, between 23 and 34% were highly satisfied; for those age 50 and over only between 6.45 and 14.29% had the same sentiment. About a quarter of untenured faculty were highly satisfied while only 6.82% of tenured faculty felt the same way. Medical school faculty were much happier than those in other schools or faculties; 27.66% of medical school faculty were highly satisfied vs only 16.13% of those in biology faculties, 7.69% of those in chemistry faculties and none in schools of public health, nursing or medical informatics.

Level of Satisfaction with Medical or Life Sciences General Quality of Library Assistance to Patrons

We also asked about the quality of library assistance to patrons, querying: how satisfied are you? Is help there when you need it? Satisfaction levels were high in this respect with 27.59% highly satisfied and 34.48% satisfied; 10.92% were somewhat satisfied and 0.57% were respectively dissatisfied and highly dissatisfied. Satisfaction was particularly high in Australia/New Zealand with 50% highly satisfied and another 40% satisfied. Scholars at private universities and those under age 40 were more satisfied than others with their library's level of service and provisions for help to library patrons.

Level of Satisfaction with Medical or Life Sciences Library General Level of Physical Comfort for Patrons

Satisfaction with the level of physical comfort in the library was somewhat less pronounced though mostly positive. 20.69% of those surveyed were highly satisfied and 34.48% satisfied. 11.49% were merely somewhat satisfied and 1.15% dissatisfied; 0.57% were highly dissatisfied. Canadian scholars were particularly satisfied with the level of physical comfort in their libraries with nearly 86% being highly satisfied or satisfied. Men were in general happier than women; nearly 25% of men were highly satisfied vs only 15.07% of women.

Level of Satisfaction with Medical or Life Sciences Library Skill in Training Students in Research Skills

Satisfaction was more attenuated with the library's skill in training students in research skills. 41.38% did not answer this question; only 13.22% were highly satisfied and 29.89%, satisfied, while 12.07% were only somewhat satisfied and 2.87% dissatisfied; 0,57% were dissatisfied. Canadians were much more satisfied than others; 28.57% were highly satisfied and 43.86% satisfied.

Level of Satisfaction with Medical or Life Sciences Library General Reference Services

Satisfaction with general reference services was also mixed with only 20.69% highly satisfied, though 38.51% were satisfied and only 9.2% somewhat satisfied. The more highly ranked universities, as well as private universities, were more likely than their peers to be highly satisfied with general reference services. Also, nearly 24% of men but only 16.44% of women were highly satisfied.

Level of Satisfaction with Medical or Life Sciences Library Information Technology

21.48% were highly satisfied with the quality of the library's information technology and 37.93% were satisfied; 10.992% were somewhat satisfied while none were dissatisfied and 1.15% highly dissatisfied. Only 10% in Australia/New Zealand were highly satisfied though 70% were satisfied. Once again satisfaction was much higher at the more highly ranked universities; those in the bottom quartile in the sample had only 12.2% express a high-level of satisfaction vs about 27.3% to 29.55% of those in top two quartiles. Men were in general easier to please than women; nearly 26% of the men were highly satisfied with the library's information technology vs. only 16.44% of women.

How the Medical or Life Science Library Fares Compared with Other Departments and Services of the University

We asked: Compared to other services and departments connected to the life sciences faculty at your university the library is generally less efficient, as efficient or more efficient? In general, the libraries fared well. Only 4.02% thought the library less efficient than other services, while 23% considered it more efficient and 59.77%, as efficient. 13.22% did not answer the question.

The Darwinian World of the Medical & other Life Sciences Libraries

In general, library satisfaction levels seem much more highly correlated with world university rankings in medicine and other life sciences than in other academic fields. It is possible that the more highly ranked institutions enjoy higher levels of funding than those ranked lower and that in medicine and life sciences, with the general high cost of journals and other inputs in the scientific process, that the cost of excellence is simply greater than in other fields. Consequently, the best funded universities - and their libraries - enjoy an advantage in this area that simply does not mean as much, or perhaps nothing at all - in academic fields in which the inputs, scholarly information and others, are less expensive.

It even seems likely that the very high cost of all things medical in the United States, has pushed up the world price level for all medical and related life sciences inputs, so that all are affected, even not for profit educational institutions, even those outside the United States, as all are competing for, and bidding for, the same type of resources. No pun intended, but the medical and life sciences library world seems more Darwinian than other academic library worlds.

What do you most like about the scientific and scholarly resources of your academic or medical library?

Tenured

1) Online resources.
2) online access
3) most readily accessible and librarian helpful
4) Best on-line journal availability of any university I've attended or worked at
5) Quiet space
6) Multidisciplinary Online accessibility
7) helpful, accessible
8) digitized library
9) access to books and journals online
10) High caliber of science and ease of collaboration
11) I rarely use it
12) online access
13) online services
14) Access to online journals.
15) Excellent staff. Adequate collection. Excellent interlibrary loan program.
16) Quick turnaround on inter library loan requests
17) online access
18) Not using it at all
19) excellent coverage of the important scholarly journals
20) Subscriptions to many journals and software tools.
21) staff
22) Extensive journal and search engine subscriptions
23) Nothing in particular
24) avalability
25) Broad availability
26) Good staff and resources
27) Ease of electronic access to peer-reviewed and other literature.
28) the availability of online resources
29) easy access to electronic journals or inter-library loan; reference librarian services
30) The staff
31) lots of online and physical resources
32) Online access directly or via interlibrary loan to almost any journal article on the planet
33) Completeness of resources, excellence of librarians, excellence of physical facilities
34) online access
35) Online access.
36) Excellent online access to materials; Excellent librarian assistance
37) Helpfulness of staff; Availability of e-resources

Not tenured but on a tenure track

1) Very helpful staff. Iliad makes getting any article possible and is quick.
2) access to Medline and e-journals
3) Easy to get the full papers.
4) Good internet-based resources.
5) I do not use the library
6) Institution has many subscriptions to scholarly journals
7) Online journal
8) I like that I can visit it online and that many things are e-books.
9) Online access.
10) Access to a wide range of academic journals.
11) Good access to medical journals electronically
12) ability to get any information even if have to buy from other institutions (a journal they do not purchase)
13) online access to most journals I require, and then responsive interlibrary loan resources for others
14) online options and availability of personnel
15) Easily accessible
16) interlibrary loan

Not tenured and not on a tenure track

1) the online paper library
2) library
3) Online literature access
4) Access to nearly any reference
5) Ease of access to professional scientific journals and electronic access at or away from campus to desired scientific primary literature
6) Many journal subscriptions
7) Digital library
8) They are large, spacious, contain a lot of resources
9) Satisfied
10) Online access available
11) Ease of access through internet
12) Ease of use and broad selection. Very little is unavailable.
13) Available all times.
14) Environment, equipment
15) Online access
16) Full text accessibility of many journals and textbooks
17) Most scholarly journals are available electronically.
18) they're good and well-kept-up
19) Easily access
20) Library

21) It has many journals and can get any paper that you want in maximum two weeks.
22) Availability of quick access to journals
23) online library pubmed access
24) Online availability of its resources
25) Good academic journal subscriptions. Faculty members (which I consider to be a scholarly resource) provide good scientific exchange and make for a positive work environment.
26) large collectiion
27) Most journals are accessible through the University online system
28) very good staff in library
29) We have nearly everything available to us in electronic format
30) Shared Lab spaces
31) Easy to access and the availability of the librarians
32) They have online copies to most issues and support staff in many ways.
33) n/a
34) Easy to access over internet to, and simple procedures to request for, almost all publications in need
35) Learn more biological knowledge.
36) Robust collection. Librarians there to help
37) Good electronic access
38) Comprehensive access to numerous journals
39) online access to publications
40) It's open
41) Interlibrary loan is easy. Library e-resources are excellent.
42) on line
43) Size and accessibility
44) remote access
45) On site; Easily accessible; Knowledgeable help
46) Library resources example BrowZine
47) Easy to access and has multiple options
48) We have a decent selection of journal subscriptions
49) I have not had a chance to explore it yet
50) Remote access to books/ journals
51) e-access
52) online access to databases and journal publications
53) availability of resources online; direct link to library/full-text from sources such as PubMed
54) Availability of services like endnote, up-to-date, and almost all significant scientific journals online
55) easy access to materials. Quiet study/reading environment
56) ease of use and availability

57) broad range of talented people
58) Helpful, accessible, much of what you need online
59) Electronic access. Great services. I don’t' need to visit the library...all on line.
60) No comment
61) Extensive library of resources makes finding relevant research material highly accessible
62) On-line access; Most resources are available
63) Ease of online access and acquirement of journal articles and books; ability to access across hundreds of journals in various unrelated fields
64) availability of resource and experts in subject
65) available on line
66) Don't have one on-site
67) electronic access

University does not offer tenure

1) Virtual library, online journal access.
2) Huge range of resources available, with most accessible online.
3) many journals are available online
4) Excellent electronic access

What do you least like about your academic or medical library's scientific and scholarly resources?

Tenured

1) Faster connection to pdf files.
2) no access to nature journals
3) Enormous number of journals and books available on line through the U of M library system
4) lack of access to journals
5) Not centrally located to all the health sciences. resources are fragmented.
6) No complaints there
7) some limitations in journals available
8) Reduction of Funding
9) Although I have no need to use it, the physical medical library space is a little dull and uninviting.
10) N/A
11) Limited journal electronic access
12) limited journals available
13) Inadequate
14) Massive budget but they do not provide critical software
15) Many journals are not available for on-line access unless you use Interlibrary Loan
16) most online
17) Good research librarians
18) some of the journals I would like are not in the collection
19) Some journals are not available
20) nothing
21) have to connect via VPN to get full texts to show up off campus; often slow and cumbersome
22) The same
23) when they only have abstracts and library hasn't paid full fees for full access

Not tenured but on a tenure track

1) Subscriptions *seem* to change frequently.
2) doesn't have access to all the journals I want
3) Limited access to some journals (full paper down load).
4) A few select journals are not available.
5) I do not use the library
6) Have to login through the university library to access said journals, even when on campus and connected to the network.
7) N/A
8) There was a paper I needed two days ago and we didn't have it. I could've requested it, but honestly was too lazy to fill out the form.

9) The physical science library is rather far from my building.
10) Limited access to journals in my field (cognitive psychology/neuroscience)
11) number of immediate access articles I have is not ideal - less than I would like
12) ILL required for more journals than I would like
13) Lacking access to some journals
14) Our library is now mostly digital with few books or librarians available

Not tenured and not on a tenure track

1) no library in our CREC center
2) computer
3) online journal access
4) It can take a few days to order a book or to order a scanned copy of a book chapter
5) Time and ability to obtain articles not presently archived
6) nothing
7) there are not enough journal subscriptions
8) More e-journal resources
9) Lack of access to many of the medical journals. Books at a centralized location that is far and inability to browse through books.
10) it seems adequate if not very good
11) That everything is not available.
12) focus is on grad students not postdocs
13) Inadequate journal holdings, not enough titles
14) Some of the textbooks do not provide online versions
15) Electronic books are take too many clicks to access.
16) Poor interaction/mentoring
17) The number of paper journals is decreasing.
18) Most of these library resources on the medical campus, which lies on the other side of a 1,371-acre park.
19) Terrible electronic access to full text--Bad interface and major problems with downloading full text
20) Most of the non-electronic resources were removed to "update" the medical library
21) temperature control, lack of privacy
22) Not applicable.
23) n/a
24) Core facilities
25) No other bioinformatic fellow to communicate with.
26) Physical location is not close to my clinical site
27) No books
28) Access to materials off campus is a cumbersome process
29) continual reduction in the number of journals we have access to
30) The full-text article is hard to access with Endnote

31) Not good at record keeping on individuals (have claimed for years I never returned a book that I did return).
32) Size and accessibility
33) lots of subscriptions
34) Na
35) We could have a lot more journal subscriptions to veterinary specific research journals and human medical journals
36) I have not had a chance to explore it yet
37) limited online access due to the limited library funds for online subscriptions
38) none
39) It's a bit far from my academic office, and will be even further in the new clinical building.
40) ???
41) immense size is isolating
42) n/a
43) Proposal consulting service
44) Large compilation, so organization/search parameters could be altered to make searching for relevant literature more user friendly (i.e. categorize as field based rather than just alphabetical)
45) Nil
46) Must re-enter login information for every journal accessed. It would be better if I could just log in once per session and not have to keep entering my username/password for every different journal b/c I frequently need several articles at a time
47) limited budget due to number of individuals competing for research funds
48) distance

University does not offer tenure

1) n/a

Table 1.1 How many times did you personally visit your academic or medical library in the past 30 days?

	Mean	Median	Minimum	Maximum
Entire sample	2.22	0.00	0.00	50.00

Table 1.2 How many times did you personally visit your academic or medical library in the past 30 days? Broken out by country

Country	Mean	Median	Minimum	Maximum
USA	1.90	0.00	0.00	30.00
Canada	7.29	0.00	0.00	50.00
UK/Ireland	1.05	0.00	0.00	10.00
Australia/New Zealand	4.00	1.00	0.00	30.00

Table 1.3 How many times did you personally visit your academic or medical library in the past 30 days? Broken out by US News and World Report World Ranking

US News and World Report World Ranking	Mean	Median	Minimum	Maximum
Less than 26	1.52	0.00	0.00	30.00
26 - 90	1.60	0.00	0.00	30.00
91 - 135	1.70	0.00	0.00	30.00
More than 135	3.76	1.00	0.00	50.00

Table 1.4 How many times did you personally visit your academic or medical library in the past 30 days? Broken out by annual tuition

Annual tuition, $	Mean	Median	Minimum	Maximum
Less than 14500	1.86	0.00	0.00	30.00
14500 - 29500	2.25	0.00	0.00	30.00
29501 - 45500	1.78	1.00	0.00	30.00
More than 45500	2.97	0.00	0.00	50.00

Table 1.5 How many times did you personally visit your academic or medical library in the past 30 days? Broken out by public and private status

Public and private status	Mean	Median	Minimum	Maximum
Public	2.27	0.00	0.00	50.00
Private	2.11	0.00	0.00	30.00

Table 1.6 How many times did you personally visit your academic or medical library in the past 30 days? Broken out by gender of the survey participant

You are male or female?	Mean	Median	Minimum	Maximum
Male	2.36	0.00	0.00	50.00
Female	2.06	0.50	0.00	30.00

Table 1.7 How many times did you personally visit your academic or medical library in the past 30 days? Broken out by FTE

FTE	Mean	Median	Minimum	Maximum
Less than 8000	2.08	0.00	0.00	30.00
8000 - 16000	1.56	0.00	0.00	30.00
16001 - 35500	2.49	0.00	0.00	30.00
More than 35500	2.74	0.00	0.00	50.00

Table 1.8 How many times did you personally visit your academic or medical library in the past 30 days? Broken out by age range of the survey participant

Which age band best describes you:	Mean	Median	Minimum	Maximum
30 or Under	1.00	0.00	0.00	6.00
31 - 39	2.95	0.00	0.00	30.00
40 - 49	1.70	0.00	0.00	30.00
50 - 59	3.07	1.00	0.00	50.00
60 or over	1.33	0.00	0.00	14.00

Table 1.9 How many times did you personally visit your academic or medical library in the past 30 days? Broken out by tenure status

Tenure status	Mean	Median	Minimum	Maximum
Tenured	1.72	0.00	0.00	30.00
Not tenured but on a tenure track	2.47	0.00	0.00	30.00
Not tenured and not on a tenure track	2.50	0.00	0.00	50.00
University does not offer tenure	0.80	1.00	0.00	2.00

Table 1.10 How many times did you personally visit your academic or medical library in the past 30 days? Broken out by academic title of the survey participant

Which phrase best describes your role or title at your university?	Mean	Median	Minimum	Maximum
Professor	0.48	0.00	0.00	2.00
Associate Professor or Reader	1.04	1.00	0.00	5.00
Assistant Professor	1.91	0.00	0.00	30.00
Lecturer or Instructor	7.00	4.00	0.00	30.00
Postdoc or Fellow	3.43	0.00	0.00	50.00

Table 1.11 How many times did you personally visit your academic or medical library in the past 30 days? Broken out by school or academic department of the survey participant

Which phrase best describes your academic department?	Mean	Median	Minimum	Maximum
Medical School Department	2.36	0.00	0.00	50.00
University Faculty of Biology	0.76	0.00	0.00	6.00
University Faculty of Chemistry	4.25	0.00	0.00	30.00
Department or School of Public Health, Nursing, Healthcare Informatics	2.72	1.00	0.00	30.00
Dentistry	0.33	0.00	0.00	1.00
Veterinary	1.50	1.00	0.00	4.00

Table 2 How satisfied are you with your academic library's services in the following areas?

Table 2.1.1 How satisfied are you with your academic library's Inter-library loan services?

	No Answer	Highly Satisfied	Satisfied	Somewhat Satisfied	Dissatisfied	Highly Dissatisfied
Entire sample	32.18%	24.14%	35.63%	6.90%	1.15%	0.00%

Table 2.1.2 How satisfied are you with your academic library's Inter-library loan services? Broken out by country

Country	No Answer	Highly Satisfied	Satisfied	Somewhat Satisfied	Dissatisfied	Highly Dissatisfied
USA	32.58%	26.52%	32.58%	6.82%	1.52%	0.00%
Canada	28.57%	28.57%	28.57%	14.29%	0.00%	0.00%
UK/Ireland	40.00%	8.00%	44.00%	8.00%	0.00%	0.00%
Australia/New Zealand	10.00%	30.00%	60.00%	0.00%	0.00%	0.00%

Table 2.1.3 How satisfied are you with your academic library's Inter-library loan services? Broken out by US News and World Report World Ranking

US News and World Report World Ranking	No Answer	Highly Satisfied	Satisfied	Somewhat Satisfied	Dissatisfied	Highly Dissatisfied
Less than 25	31.82%	34.09%	27.27%	6.82%	0.00%	0.00%
26 - 90	34.09%	20.45%	36.36%	6.82%	2.27%	0.00%
91 - 135	46.67%	17.78%	28.89%	4.44%	2.22%	0.00%
More than 135	14.63%	24.39%	51.22%	9.76%	0.00%	0.00%

Table 2.1.4 How satisfied are you with your academic library's Inter-library loan services? Broken out by annual tuition

Annual tuition, $	No Answer	Highly Satisfied	Satisfied	Somewhat Satisfied	Dissatisfied	Highly Dissatisfied
Less than 14500	37.78%	11.11%	42.22%	8.89%	0.00%	0.00%
14500 - 29500	30.23%	18.60%	39.53%	9.30%	2.33%	0.00%
29501 - 45500	22.73%	43.18%	29.55%	2.27%	2.27%	0.00%
More than 45500	38.10%	23.81%	30.95%	7.14%	0.00%	0.00%

Table 2.1.5 How satisfied are you with your academic library's Inter-library loan services? Broken out by public and private status

Public and private status	No Answer	Highly Satisfied	Satisfied	Somewhat Satisfied	Dissatisfied	Highly Dissatisfied
Public	33.91%	17.39%	40.00%	7.83%	0.87%	0.00%
Private	28.81%	37.29%	27.12%	5.08%	1.69%	0.00%

Table 2.1.6 How satisfied are you with your academic library's Inter-library loan services? Broken out by gender of the survey participant

You are male or female?	No Answer	Highly Satisfied	Satisfied	Somewhat Satisfied	Dissatisfied	Highly Dissatisfied
Male	31.68%	25.74%	36.63%	5.94%	0.00%	0.00%
Female	32.88%	21.92%	34.25%	8.22%	2.74%	0.00%

Table 2.1.7 How satisfied are you with your academic library's Inter-library loan services? Broken out by FTE

FTE	No Answer	Highly Satisfied	Satisfied	Somewhat Satisfied	Dissatisfied	Highly Dissatisfied
Less than 8000	35.71%	19.05%	35.71%	7.14%	2.38%	0.00%
8000 - 16000	33.33%	37.78%	22.22%	4.44%	2.22%	0.00%
16001 - 35500	27.27%	15.91%	50.00%	6.82%	0.00%	0.00%
More than 35500	32.56%	23.26%	34.88%	9.30%	0.00%	0.00%

Table 2.1.8 How satisfied are you with your academic library's Inter-library loan services? Broken out by age range of the survey participant

Which age band best describes you:	No Answer	Highly Satisfied	Satisfied	Somewhat Satisfied	Dissatisfied	Highly Dissatisfied
30 or Under	53.85%	11.54%	34.62%	0.00%	0.00%	0.00%
31 - 39	33.96%	30.19%	22.64%	9.43%	3.77%	0.00%
40 - 49	22.22%	27.78%	44.44%	5.56%	0.00%	0.00%
50 - 59	29.03%	25.81%	35.48%	9.68%	0.00%	0.00%
60 or over	25.00%	17.86%	50.00%	7.14%	0.00%	0.00%

Table 2.1.9 How satisfied are you with your academic library's Inter-library loan services? Broken out by tenure status

Tenure status	No Answer	Highly Satisfied	Satisfied	Somewhat Satisfied	Dissatisfied	Highly Dissatisfied
Tenured	20.45%	15.91%	52.27%	11.36%	0.00%	0.00%
Not tenured but on a tenure track	38.10%	28.57%	23.81%	9.52%	0.00%	0.00%
Not tenured and not on a tenure track	37.25%	25.49%	31.37%	3.92%	1.96%	0.00%
University does not offer tenure	14.29%	42.86%	28.57%	14.29%	0.00%	0.00%

Table 2.1.10 How satisfied are you with your academic library's Inter-library loan services? Broken out by academic title of the survey participant

Which phrase best describes your role or title at your university?	No Answer	Highly Satisfied	Satisfied	Somewhat Satisfied	Dissatisfied	Highly Dissatisfied
Professor	28.57%	22.86%	40.00%	8.57%	0.00%	0.00%
Associate Professor or Reader	3.85%	23.08%	65.38%	7.69%	0.00%	0.00%
Assistant Professor	35.71%	23.81%	30.95%	7.14%	2.38%	0.00%
Lecturer or Instructor	33.33%	11.11%	44.44%	11.11%	0.00%	0.00%
Postdoc or Fellow	43.55%	27.42%	22.58%	4.84%	1.61%	0.00%

Table 2.1.11 How satisfied are you with your academic library's Inter-library loan services? Broken out by school or academic department of the survey participant

Which phrase best describes your academic department?	No Answer	Highly Satisfied	Satisfied	Somewhat Satisfied	Dissatisfied	Highly Dissatisfied
Medical School Department	30.85%	35.11%	26.60%	6.38%	1.06%	0.00%
University Faculty of Biology	51.61%	6.45%	32.26%	6.45%	3.23%	0.00%
University Faculty of Chemistry	46.15%	7.69%	38.46%	7.69%	0.00%	0.00%
Department or School of Public Health, Nursing, Healthcare Informatics	7.41%	18.52%	66.67%	7.41%	0.00%	0.00%
Dentistry	60.00%	0.00%	20.00%	20.00%	0.00%	0.00%
Veterinary	0.00%	25.00%	75.00%	0.00%	0.00%	0.00%

Table 2.2.1 How satisfied are you with your academic library's eBook collection and services?

	No Answer	Highly Satisfied	Satisfied	Somewhat Satisfied	Dissatisfied	Highly Dissatisfied
Entire sample	26.44%	21.26%	39.08%	10.92%	2.30%	0.00%

Table 2.2.2 How satisfied are you with your academic library's eBook collection and services? Broken out by country

Country	No Answer	Highly Satisfied	Satisfied	Somewhat Satisfied	Dissatisfied	Highly Dissatisfied
USA	27.27%	23.48%	39.39%	7.58%	2.27%	0.00%
Canada	0.00%	14.29%	71.43%	14.29%	0.00%	0.00%
UK/Ireland	36.00%	12.00%	28.00%	20.00%	4.00%	0.00%
Australia/New Zealand	10.00%	20.00%	40.00%	30.00%	0.00%	0.00%

Table 2.2.3 How satisfied are you with your academic library's eBook collection and services? Broken out by US News and World Report World Ranking

US News and World Report World Ranking	No Answer	Highly Satisfied	Satisfied	Somewhat Satisfied	Dissatisfied	Highly Dissatisfied
Less than 25	25.00%	27.27%	38.64%	6.82%	2.27%	0.00%
26 - 90	15.91%	34.09%	36.36%	11.36%	2.27%	0.00%
91 - 135	40.00%	17.78%	40.00%	0.00%	2.22%	0.00%
More than 135	24.39%	4.88%	41.46%	26.83%	2.44%	0.00%

Table 2.2.4 How satisfied are you with your academic library's eBook collection and services? Broken out by annual tuition

Annual tuition, $	No Answer	Highly Satisfied	Satisfied	Somewhat Satisfied	Dissatisfied	Highly Dissatisfied
Less than 14500	31.11%	8.89%	40.00%	17.78%	2.22%	0.00%
14500 - 29500	30.23%	16.28%	41.86%	6.98%	4.65%	0.00%
29501 - 45500	20.45%	34.09%	31.82%	13.64%	0.00%	0.00%
More than 45500	23.81%	26.19%	42.86%	4.76%	2.38%	0.00%

Table 2.2.5 How satisfied are you with your academic library's eBook collection and services? Broken out by public and private status

Public and private status	No Answer	Highly Satisfied	Satisfied	Somewhat Satisfied	Dissatisfied	Highly Dissatisfied
Public	29.57%	16.52%	39.13%	12.17%	2.61%	0.00%
Private	20.34%	30.51%	38.98%	8.47%	1.69%	0.00%

Table 2.2.6 How satisfied are you with your academic library's eBook collection and services? Broken out by gender of the survey participant

You are male or female?	No Answer	Highly Satisfied	Satisfied	Somewhat Satisfied	Dissatisfied	Highly Dissatisfied
Male	26.73%	21.78%	39.60%	10.89%	0.99%	0.00%
Female	26.03%	20.55%	38.36%	10.96%	4.11%	0.00%

Table 2.2.7 How satisfied are you with your academic library's eBook collection and services? Broken out by FTE

FTE	No Answer	Highly Satisfied	Satisfied	Somewhat Satisfied	Dissatisfied	Highly Dissatisfied
Less than 8000	33.33%	16.67%	38.10%	7.14%	4.76%	0.00%
8000 - 16000	24.44%	33.33%	33.33%	6.67%	2.22%	0.00%
16001 - 35500	25.00%	15.91%	45.45%	13.64%	0.00%	0.00%
More than 35500	23.26%	18.60%	39.53%	16.28%	2.33%	0.00%

Table 2.2.8 How satisfied are you with your academic library's eBook collection and services? Broken out by age range of the survey participant

Which age band best describes you?	No Answer	Highly Satisfied	Satisfied	Somewhat Satisfied	Dissatisfied	Highly Dissatisfied
30 or Under	34.62%	19.23%	38.46%	3.85%	3.85%	0.00%
31 - 39	18.87%	32.08%	32.08%	13.21%	3.77%	0.00%
40 - 49	33.33%	16.67%	41.67%	8.33%	0.00%	0.00%
50 - 59	25.81%	12.90%	38.71%	19.35%	3.23%	0.00%
60 or over	25.00%	17.86%	50.00%	7.14%	0.00%	0.00%

Table 2.2.9 How satisfied are you with your academic library's eBook collection and services? Broken out by tenure status

Tenure status	No Answer	Highly Satisfied	Satisfied	Somewhat Satisfied	Dissatisfied	Highly Dissatisfied
Tenured	20.45%	11.36%	47.73%	20.45%	0.00%	0.00%
Not tenured but on a tenure track	28.57%	19.05%	47.62%	4.76%	0.00%	0.00%
Not tenured and not on a tenure track	28.43%	25.49%	36.27%	5.88%	3.92%	0.00%
University does not offer tenure	28.57%	28.57%	0.00%	42.86%	0.00%	0.00%

Table 2.2.10 How satisfied are you with your academic library's eBook collection and services? Broken out by academic title of the survey participant

Which phrase best describes your role or title at your university?	No Answer	Highly Satisfied	Satisfied	Somewhat Satisfied	Dissatisfied	Highly Dissatisfied
Professor	25.71%	20.00%	42.86%	11.43%	0.00%	0.00%
Associate Professor or Reader	11.54%	11.54%	53.85%	19.23%	3.85%	0.00%
Assistant Professor	28.57%	16.67%	42.86%	9.52%	2.38%	0.00%
Lecturer or Instructor	22.22%	11.11%	55.56%	11.11%	0.00%	0.00%
Postdoc or Fellow	32.26%	30.65%	25.81%	8.06%	3.23%	0.00%

Table 2.2.11 How satisfied are you with your academic library's eBook collection and services? Broken out by school or academic department of the survey participant

Which phrase best describes your academic department?	No Answer	Highly Satisfied	Satisfied	Somewhat Satisfied	Dissatisfied	Highly Dissatisfied
Medical School Department	26.60%	29.79%	36.17%	6.38%	1.06%	0.00%
University Faculty of Biology	45.16%	12.90%	29.03%	9.68%	3.23%	0.00%
University Faculty of Chemistry	15.38%	15.38%	46.15%	23.08%	0.00%	0.00%
Department or School of Public Health, Nursing, Healthcare Informatics	11.11%	3.70%	55.56%	22.22%	7.41%	0.00%
Dentistry	20.00%	20.00%	40.00%	20.00%	0.00%	0.00%
Veterinary	25.00%	25.00%	50.00%	0.00%	0.00%	0.00%

Table 2.3.1 How satisfied are you with the level of knowledge of your field of the library's subject specialists

	No Answer	Highly Satisfied	Satisfied	Somewhat Satisfied	Dissatisfied	Highly Dissatisfied
Entire sample	39.08%	16.67%	30.46%	11.49%	1.72%	0.57%

Table 2.3.2 How satisfied are you with the level of knowledge of your field of the library's subject specialists Broken out by country

Country	No Answer	Highly Satisfied	Satisfied	Somewhat Satisfied	Dissatisfied	Highly Dissatisfied
USA	39.39%	18.18%	28.03%	12.12%	1.52%	0.76%
Canada	28.57%	14.29%	42.86%	0.00%	14.29%	0.00%
UK/Ireland	44.00%	12.00%	32.00%	12.00%	0.00%	0.00%
Australia/New Zealand	30.00%	10.00%	50.00%	10.00%	0.00%	0.00%

Table 2.3.3 How satisfied are you with the level of knowledge of your field of the library's subject specialists Broken out by US News and World Report World Ranking

US News and World Report World Ranking	No Answer	Highly Satisfied	Satisfied	Somewhat Satisfied	Dissatisfied	Highly Dissatisfied
Less than 25	34.09%	27.27%	27.27%	9.09%	0.00%	2.27%
26 - 90	38.64%	20.45%	27.27%	13.64%	0.00%	0.00%
91 - 135	53.33%	11.11%	26.67%	6.67%	2.22%	0.00%
More than 135	29.27%	7.32%	41.46%	17.07%	4.88%	0.00%

Table 2.3.4 How satisfied are you with the level of knowledge of your field of the library's subject specialists Broken out by annual tuition, $

Annual tuition, $	No Answer	Highly Satisfied	Satisfied	Somewhat Satisfied	Dissatisfied	Highly Dissatisfied
Less than 14500	44.44%	6.67%	35.56%	8.89%	4.44%	0.00%
14500 - 29500	44.19%	9.30%	37.21%	9.30%	0.00%	0.00%
29501 - 45500	27.27%	29.55%	25.00%	13.64%	2.27%	2.27%
More than 45500	40.48%	21.43%	23.81%	14.29%	0.00%	0.00%

Table 2.3.5 How satisfied are you with the level of knowledge of your field of the library's subject specialists Broken out by public and private status

Public and private status	No Answer	Highly Satisfied	Satisfied	Somewhat Satisfied	Dissatisfied	Highly Dissatisfied
Public	40.87%	13.04%	33.91%	9.57%	1.74%	0.87%
Private	35.59%	23.73%	23.73%	15.25%	1.69%	0.00%

Table 2.3.6 How satisfied are you with the level of knowledge of your field of the library's subject specialists Broken out by gender of the survey participant

You are male or female?	No Answer	Highly Satisfied	Satisfied	Somewhat Satisfied	Dissatisfied	Highly Dissatisfied
Male	36.63%	18.81%	30.69%	13.86%	0.00%	0.00%
Female	42.47%	13.70%	30.14%	8.22%	4.11%	1.37%

Table 2.3.7 How satisfied are you with the level of knowledge of your field of the library's subject specialists Broken out by FTE

FTE	No Answer	Highly Satisfied	Satisfied	Somewhat Satisfied	Dissatisfied	Highly Dissatisfied
Less than 8000	40.48%	14.29%	28.57%	11.90%	4.76%	0.00%
8000 - 16000	40.00%	26.67%	22.22%	11.11%	0.00%	0.00%
16001 - 35500	40.91%	6.82%	38.64%	13.64%	0.00%	0.00%
More than 35500	34.88%	18.60%	32.56%	9.30%	2.33%	2.33%

Table 2.3.8 How satisfied are you with the level of knowledge of your field of the library's subject specialists Broken out by age range of the survey participant

Which age band best describes you?	No Answer	Highly Satisfied	Satisfied	Somewhat Satisfied	Dissatisfied	Highly Dissatisfied
30 or Under	46.15%	15.38%	34.62%	3.85%	0.00%	0.00%
31 - 39	41.51%	24.53%	15.09%	16.98%	0.00%	1.89%
40 - 49	38.89%	8.33%	38.89%	11.11%	2.78%	0.00%
50 - 59	35.48%	9.68%	35.48%	12.90%	6.45%	0.00%
60 or over	32.14%	21.43%	39.29%	7.14%	0.00%	0.00%

Table 2.3.9 How satisfied are you with the level of knowledge of your field of the library's subject specialists Broken out by tenure status

Tenure status	No Answer	Highly Satisfied	Satisfied	Somewhat Satisfied	Dissatisfied	Highly Dissatisfied
Tenured	20.45%	13.64%	47.73%	15.91%	2.27%	0.00%
Not tenured but on a tenure track	57.14%	14.29%	14.29%	9.52%	4.76%	0.00%
Not tenured and not on a tenure track	42.16%	19.61%	26.47%	9.80%	0.98%	0.98%
University does not offer tenure	57.14%	0.00%	28.57%	14.29%	0.00%	0.00%

Table 2.3.10 How satisfied are you with the level of knowledge of your field of the library's subject specialists Broken out by academic title of the survey participant

Which phrase best describes your role or title at your university?	No Answer	Highly Satisfied	Satisfied	Somewhat Satisfied	Dissatisfied	Highly Dissatisfied
Professor	28.57%	22.86%	34.29%	11.43%	2.86%	0.00%
Associate Professor or Reader	23.08%	3.85%	50.00%	15.38%	7.69%	0.00%
Assistant Professor	59.52%	9.52%	19.05%	11.90%	0.00%	0.00%
Lecturer or Instructor	44.44%	11.11%	44.44%	0.00%	0.00%	0.00%
Postdoc or Fellow	37.10%	24.19%	25.81%	11.29%	0.00%	1.61%

Table 2.3.11 How satisfied are you with the level of knowledge of your field of the library's subject specialists Broken out by school or academic department of the survey participant

Which phrase best describes your academic department?	No Answer	Highly Satisfied	Satisfied	Somewhat Satisfied	Dissatisfied	Highly Dissatisfied
Medical School Department	43.62%	18.09%	24.47%	11.70%	1.06%	1.06%
University Faculty of Biology	48.39%	16.13%	19.35%	12.90%	3.23%	0.00%
University Faculty of Chemistry	38.46%	7.69%	38.46%	15.38%	0.00%	0.00%
Department or School of Public Health, Nursing, Healthcare Informatics	18.52%	11.11%	59.26%	11.11%	0.00%	0.00%
Dentistry	40.00%	40.00%	0.00%	0.00%	20.00%	0.00%
Veterinary	0.00%	25.00%	75.00%	0.00%	0.00%	0.00%

Table 2.4.1 How satisfied are you with the quality and range of databases made available to you?

	No Answer	Highly Satisfied	Satisfied	Somewhat Satisfied	Dissatisfied	Highly Dissatisfied
Entire sample	14.94%	35.06%	37.36%	9.20%	1.72%	1.72%

Table 2.4.2 How satisfied are you with the quality and range of databases made available to you? Broken out by country

Country	No Answer	Highly Satisfied	Satisfied	Somewhat Satisfied	Dissatisfied	Highly Dissatisfied
USA	16.67%	37.12%	33.33%	9.09%	1.52%	2.27%
Canada	0.00%	14.29%	57.14%	28.57%	0.00%	0.00%
UK/Ireland	16.00%	24.00%	52.00%	8.00%	0.00%	0.00%
Australia/New Zealand	0.00%	50.00%	40.00%	0.00%	10.00%	0.00%

Table 2.4.3 How satisfied are you with the quality and range of databases made available to you? Broken out by US News and World Report World Ranking

US News and World Report World Ranking	No Answer	Highly Satisfied	Satisfied	Somewhat Satisfied	Dissatisfied	Highly Dissatisfied
Less than 25	13.64%	40.91%	34.09%	9.09%	0.00%	2.27%
26 - 90	9.09%	47.73%	29.55%	9.09%	0.00%	4.55%
91 - 135	28.89%	28.89%	33.33%	4.44%	4.44%	0.00%
More than 135	7.32%	21.95%	53.66%	14.63%	2.44%	0.00%

Table 2.4.4 How satisfied are you with the quality and range of databases made available to you? Broken out by annual tuition

Annual tuition, $	No Answer	Highly Satisfied	Satisfied	Somewhat Satisfied	Dissatisfied	Highly Dissatisfied
Less than 14500	17.78%	26.67%	48.89%	6.67%	0.00%	0.00%
14500 - 29500	23.26%	27.91%	32.56%	9.30%	4.65%	2.33%
29501 - 45500	9.09%	45.45%	31.82%	9.09%	2.27%	2.27%
More than 45500	9.52%	40.48%	35.71%	11.90%	0.00%	2.38%

Table 2.4.5 How satisfied are you with the quality and range of databases made available to you? Broken out by public and private status

Public and private status	No Answer	Highly Satisfied	Satisfied	Somewhat Satisfied	Dissatisfied	Highly Dissatisfied
Public	17.39%	31.30%	39.13%	7.83%	2.61%	1.74%
Private	10.17%	42.37%	33.90%	11.86%	0.00%	1.69%

Table 2.4.6 How satisfied are you with the quality and range of databases made available to you? Broken out by gender of the survey participant

You are male or female?	No Answer	Highly Satisfied	Satisfied	Somewhat Satisfied	Dissatisfied	Highly Dissatisfied
Male	14.85%	35.64%	37.62%	9.90%	0.00%	1.98%
Female	15.07%	34.25%	36.99%	8.22%	4.11%	1.37%

Table 2.4.7 How satisfied are you with the quality and range of databases made available to you? Broken out by FTE

FTE	No Answer	Highly Satisfied	Satisfied	Somewhat Satisfied	Dissatisfied	Highly Dissatisfied
Less than 8000	23.81%	26.19%	33.33%	11.90%	4.76%	0.00%
8000 - 16000	11.11%	48.89%	26.67%	8.89%	0.00%	4.44%
16001 - 35500	11.36%	29.55%	52.27%	4.55%	2.27%	0.00%
More than 35500	13.95%	34.88%	37.21%	11.63%	0.00%	2.33%

Table 2.4.8 How satisfied are you with the quality and range of databases made available to you? Broken out by age range of the survey participant

Which age band best describes you:	No Answer	Highly Satisfied	Satisfied	Somewhat Satisfied	Dissatisfied	Highly Dissatisfied
30 or Under	23.08%	34.62%	34.62%	3.85%	0.00%	3.85%
31 - 39	13.21%	43.40%	30.19%	9.43%	1.89%	1.89%
40 - 49	11.11%	30.56%	44.44%	11.11%	2.78%	0.00%
50 - 59	9.68%	29.03%	41.94%	12.90%	3.23%	3.23%
60 or over	21.43%	32.14%	39.29%	7.14%	0.00%	0.00%

Table 2.4.9 How satisfied are you with the quality and range of databases made available to you? Broken out by Tenure status

Tenure status	No Answer	Highly Satisfied	Satisfied	Somewhat Satisfied	Dissatisfied	Highly Dissatisfied
Tenured	9.09%	27.27%	50.00%	11.36%	2.27%	0.00%
Not tenured but on a tenure track	9.52%	42.86%	38.10%	4.76%	4.76%	0.00%
Not tenured and not on a tenure track	18.63%	37.25%	31.37%	8.82%	0.98%	2.94%
University does not offer tenure	14.29%	28.57%	42.86%	14.29%	0.00%	0.00%

Table 2.4.10 How satisfied are you with the quality and range of databases made available to you? Broken out by academic title of the survey participant

Which phrase best describes your role or title at your university?	No Answer	Highly Satisfied	Satisfied	Somewhat Satisfied	Dissatisfied	Highly Dissatisfied
Professor	14.29%	40.00%	34.29%	8.57%	2.86%	0.00%
Associate Professor or Reader	0.00%	23.08%	57.69%	15.38%	0.00%	3.85%
Assistant Professor	16.67%	35.71%	35.71%	7.14%	4.76%	0.00%
Lecturer or Instructor	22.22%	11.11%	66.67%	0.00%	0.00%	0.00%
Postdoc or Fellow	19.35%	40.32%	27.42%	9.68%	0.00%	3.23%

Table 2.4.11 How satisfied are you with the quality and range of databases made available to you? Broken out by school or academic department of the survey participant

Which phrase best describes your academic department?	No Answer	Highly Satisfied	Satisfied	Somewhat Satisfied	Dissatisfied	Highly Dissatisfied
Medical School Department	15.96%	38.30%	32.98%	9.57%	2.13%	1.06%
University Faculty of Biology	25.81%	38.71%	25.81%	9.68%	0.00%	0.00%
University Faculty of Chemistry	7.69%	23.08%	46.15%	15.38%	0.00%	7.69%
Department or School of Public Health, Nursing, Healthcare Informatics	3.70%	22.22%	62.96%	3.70%	3.70%	3.70%
Dentistry	20.00%	40.00%	20.00%	20.00%	0.00%	0.00%
Veterinary	0.00%	50.00%	50.00%	0.00%	0.00%	0.00%

Table 2.5.1 How satisfied are you with the quality and range of the journals collection made available to you?

	No Answer	Highly Satisfied	Satisfied	Somewhat Satisfied	Dissatisfied	Highly Dissatisfied
Entire sample	12.64%	34.48%	35.06%	10.92%	6.32%	0.57%

Table 2.5.2 How satisfied are you with Broken out by country

Country	No Answer	Highly Satisfied	Satisfied	Somewhat Satisfied	Dissatisfied	Highly Dissatisfied
USA	14.39%	40.15%	31.06%	9.09%	4.55%	0.76%
Canada	0.00%	14.29%	71.43%	14.29%	0.00%	0.00%
UK/Ireland	12.00%	12.00%	48.00%	16.00%	12.00%	0.00%
Australia/New Zealand	0.00%	30.00%	30.00%	20.00%	20.00%	0.00%

Table 2.5.3 How satisfied are you with the quality and range of the journals collection made available to you? Broken out by US News and World Report World Ranking

US News and World Report World Ranking	No Answer	Highly Satisfied	Satisfied	Somewhat Satisfied	Dissatisfied	Highly Dissatisfied
Less than 25	13.64%	50.00%	29.55%	4.55%	0.00%	2.27%
26 - 90	6.82%	47.73%	36.36%	4.55%	4.55%	0.00%
91 - 135	26.67%	28.89%	31.11%	6.67%	6.67%	0.00%
More than 135	2.44%	9.76%	43.90%	29.27%	14.63%	0.00%

Table 2.5.4 How satisfied are you with the quality and range of the journals collection made available to you? Broken out by annual tuition

Annual tuition, $	No Answer	Highly Satisfied	Satisfied	Somewhat Satisfied	Dissatisfied	Highly Dissatisfied
Less than 14500	15.56%	20.00%	46.67%	11.11%	6.67%	0.00%
14500 - 29500	18.60%	25.58%	32.56%	11.63%	11.63%	0.00%
29501 - 45500	6.82%	54.55%	20.45%	9.09%	6.82%	2.27%
More than 45500	9.52%	38.10%	40.48%	11.90%	0.00%	0.00%

Table 2.5.5 How satisfied are you with the quality and range of the journals collection made available to you? Broken out by public and private status

Public and private status	No Answer	Highly Satisfied	Satisfied	Somewhat Satisfied	Dissatisfied	Highly Dissatisfied
Public	15.65%	28.70%	34.78%	12.17%	7.83%	0.87%
Private	6.78%	45.76%	35.59%	8.47%	3.39%	0.00%

Table 2.5.6 How satisfied are you with the quality and range of the journals collection made available to you? Broken out by gender of the survey participant

You are male or female?	No Answer	Highly Satisfied	Satisfied	Somewhat Satisfied	Dissatisfied	Highly Dissatisfied
Male	13.86%	35.64%	37.62%	11.88%	0.99%	0.00%
Female	10.96%	32.88%	31.51%	9.59%	13.70%	1.37%

Table 2.5.7 How satisfied are you with the quality and range of the journals collection made available to you? Broken out by FTE

FTE	No Answer	Highly Satisfied	Satisfied	Somewhat Satisfied	Dissatisfied	Highly Dissatisfied
Less than 8000	21.43%	26.19%	33.33%	7.14%	11.90%	0.00%
8000 - 16000	8.89%	53.33%	26.67%	6.67%	4.44%	0.00%
16001 - 35500	6.82%	15.91%	50.00%	20.45%	6.82%	0.00%
More than 35500	13.95%	41.86%	30.23%	9.30%	2.33%	2.33%

Table 2.5.8 How satisfied are you with the quality and range of the journals collection made available to you? Broken out by age range of the survey participant

Which age band best describes you?	No Answer	Highly Satisfied	Satisfied	Somewhat Satisfied	Dissatisfied	Highly Dissatisfied
30 or Under	23.08%	30.77%	42.31%	0.00%	3.85%	0.00%
31 - 39	11.32%	49.06%	30.19%	3.77%	3.77%	1.89%
40 - 49	8.33%	33.33%	30.56%	16.67%	11.11%	0.00%
50 - 59	6.45%	16.13%	45.16%	22.58%	9.68%	0.00%
60 or over	17.86%	32.14%	32.14%	14.29%	3.57%	0.00%

Table 2.5.9 How satisfied are you with the quality and range of the journals collection made available to you? Broken out by tenure status

Tenure status	No Answer	Highly Satisfied	Satisfied	Somewhat Satisfied	Dissatisfied	Highly Dissatisfied
Tenured	6.82%	22.73%	34.09%	27.27%	9.09%	0.00%
Not tenured but on a tenure track	4.76%	33.33%	47.62%	4.76%	9.52%	0.00%
Not tenured and not on a tenure track	16.67%	40.20%	32.35%	4.90%	4.90%	0.98%
University does not offer tenure	14.29%	28.57%	42.86%	14.29%	0.00%	0.00%

Table 2.5.10 How satisfied are you with the quality and range of the journals collection made available to you? Broken out by academic title of the survey participant

Which phrase best describes your role or title at your university?	No Answer	Highly Satisfied	Satisfied	Somewhat Satisfied	Dissatisfied	Highly Dissatisfied
Professor	11.43%	34.29%	42.86%	5.71%	5.71%	0.00%
Associate Professor or Reader	0.00%	19.23%	38.46%	30.77%	11.54%	0.00%
Assistant Professor	11.90%	26.19%	42.86%	11.90%	7.14%	0.00%
Lecturer or Instructor	22.22%	11.11%	33.33%	33.33%	0.00%	0.00%
Postdoc or Fellow	17.74%	50.00%	24.19%	1.61%	4.84%	1.61%

Table 2.5.11 How satisfied are you with the quality and range of the journals collection made available to you? Broken out by school or academic department of the survey participant

Which phrase best describes your academic department?	No Answer	Highly Satisfied	Satisfied	Somewhat Satisfied	Dissatisfied	Highly Dissatisfied
Medical School Department	13.83%	41.49%	27.66%	9.57%	6.38%	1.06%
University Faculty of Biology	19.35%	29.03%	35.48%	6.45%	9.68%	0.00%
University Faculty of Chemistry	7.69%	23.08%	53.85%	15.38%	0.00%	0.00%
Department or School of Public Health, Nursing, Healthcare Informatics	3.70%	22.22%	51.85%	14.81%	7.41%	0.00%
Dentistry	20.00%	40.00%	40.00%	0.00%	0.00%	0.00%
Veterinary	0.00%	25.00%	25.00%	50.00%	0.00%	0.00%

Table 2.6.1 How satisfied are you with your academic library's services in data curation and archiving?

	No Answer	Highly Satisfied	Satisfied	Somewhat Satisfied	Dissatisfied	Highly Dissatisfied
Entire sample	42.53%	20.11%	24.71%	9.77%	2.30%	0.57%

Table 2.6.2 How satisfied are you with your academic library's services in data curation and archiving? Broken out by country

Country	No Answer	Highly Satisfied	Satisfied	Somewhat Satisfied	Dissatisfied	Highly Dissatisfied
USA	46.97%	22.73%	19.70%	7.58%	2.27%	0.76%
Canada	42.86%	14.29%	28.57%	14.29%	0.00%	0.00%
UK/Ireland	24.00%	12.00%	44.00%	20.00%	0.00%	0.00%
Australia/New Zealand	30.00%	10.00%	40.00%	10.00%	10.00%	0.00%

Table 2.6.3 How satisfied are you with your academic library's services in data curation and archiving? Broken out by US News and World Report World Ranking

US News and World Report World Ranking	No Answer	Highly Satisfied	Satisfied	Somewhat Satisfied	Dissatisfied	Highly Dissatisfied
Less than 25	40.91%	27.27%	18.18%	9.09%	2.27%	2.27%
26 - 90	47.73%	27.27%	22.73%	2.27%	0.00%	0.00%
91 - 135	44.44%	15.56%	24.44%	13.33%	2.22%	0.00%
More than 135	36.59%	9.76%	34.15%	14.63%	4.88%	0.00%

Table 2.6.4 How satisfied are you with your academic library's services in data curation and archiving? Broken out by annual tuition

Annual tuition, $	No Answer	Highly Satisfied	Satisfied	Somewhat Satisfied	Dissatisfied	Highly Dissatisfied
Less than 14500	33.33%	11.11%	35.56%	17.78%	2.22%	0.00%
14500 - 29500	48.84%	16.28%	30.23%	4.65%	0.00%	0.00%
29501 - 45500	38.64%	34.09%	18.18%	2.27%	4.55%	2.27%
More than 45500	50.00%	19.05%	14.29%	14.29%	2.38%	0.00%

Table 2.6.5 How satisfied are you with your academic library's services in data curation and archiving? Broken out by public and private status

Public and private status	No Answer	Highly Satisfied	Satisfied	Somewhat Satisfied	Dissatisfied	Highly Dissatisfied
Public	39.13%	17.39%	28.70%	11.30%	2.61%	0.87%
Private	49.15%	25.42%	16.95%	6.78%	1.69%	0.00%

Table 2.6.6 How satisfied are you with your academic library's services in data curation and archiving? Broken out by gender of the survey participant

You are male or female?	No Answer	Highly Satisfied	Satisfied	Somewhat Satisfied	Dissatisfied	Highly Dissatisfied
Male	43.56%	19.80%	24.75%	10.89%	0.99%	0.00%
Female	41.10%	20.55%	24.66%	8.22%	4.11%	1.37%

Table 2.6.7 How satisfied are you with your academic library's services in data curation and archiving? Broken out by FTE

FTE	No Answer	Highly Satisfied	Satisfied	Somewhat Satisfied	Dissatisfied	Highly Dissatisfied
Less than 8000	42.86%	19.05%	21.43%	16.67%	0.00%	0.00%
8000 - 16000	51.11%	31.11%	13.33%	2.22%	2.22%	0.00%
16001 - 35500	38.64%	9.09%	38.64%	9.09%	4.55%	0.00%
More than 35500	37.21%	20.93%	25.58%	11.63%	2.33%	2.33%

Table 2.6.8 How satisfied are you with your academic library's services in data curation and archiving? Broken out by age range of the survey participant

Which age band best describes you?	No Answer	Highly Satisfied	Satisfied	Somewhat Satisfied	Dissatisfied	Highly Dissatisfied
30 or Under	34.62%	23.08%	38.46%	3.85%	0.00%	0.00%
31 - 39	37.74%	33.96%	15.09%	9.43%	1.89%	1.89%
40 - 49	41.67%	13.89%	36.11%	2.78%	5.56%	0.00%
50 - 59	54.84%	6.45%	16.13%	22.58%	0.00%	0.00%
60 or over	46.43%	14.29%	25.00%	10.71%	3.57%	0.00%

Table 2.6.9 How satisfied are you with your academic library's services in data curation and archiving? Broken out by Tenure status

Tenure status	No Answer	Highly Satisfied	Satisfied	Somewhat Satisfied	Dissatisfied	Highly Dissatisfied
Tenured	43.18%	6.82%	31.82%	11.36%	6.82%	0.00%
Not tenured but on a tenure track	61.90%	23.81%	9.52%	0.00%	4.76%	0.00%
Not tenured and not on a tenure track	38.24%	26.47%	23.53%	10.78%	0.00%	0.98%
University does not offer tenure	42.86%	0.00%	42.86%	14.29%	0.00%	0.00%

Table 2.6.10 How satisfied are you with your academic library's services in data curation and archiving? Broken out by academic title of the survey participant

Which phrase best describes your role or title at your university?	No Answer	Highly Satisfied	Satisfied	Somewhat Satisfied	Dissatisfied	Highly Dissatisfied
Professor	48.57%	14.29%	25.71%	5.71%	5.71%	0.00%
Associate Professor or Reader	42.31%	3.85%	26.92%	23.08%	3.85%	0.00%
Assistant Professor	54.76%	16.67%	21.43%	7.14%	0.00%	0.00%
Lecturer or Instructor	22.22%	11.11%	55.56%	0.00%	11.11%	0.00%
Postdoc or Fellow	33.87%	33.87%	20.97%	9.68%	0.00%	1.61%

Table 2.6.11 How satisfied are you with your academic library's services in data curation and archiving? Broken out by school or academic department of the survey participant

Which phrase best describes your academic department?	No Answer	Highly Satisfied	Satisfied	Somewhat Satisfied	Dissatisfied	Highly Dissatisfied
Medical School Department	43.62%	27.66%	15.96%	10.64%	1.06%	1.06%
University Faculty of Biology	45.16%	16.13%	22.58%	16.13%	0.00%	0.00%
University Faculty of Chemistry	46.15%	7.69%	46.15%	0.00%	0.00%	0.00%
Department or School of Public Health, Nursing, Healthcare Informatics	37.04%	0.00%	44.44%	7.41%	11.11%	0.00%
Dentistry	40.00%	40.00%	20.00%	0.00%	0.00%	0.00%
Veterinary	25.00%	25.00%	50.00%	0.00%	0.00%	0.00%

Table 2.7.1 How satisfied are you that help is there when you need it from the academic library staff?

	No Answer	Highly Satisfied	Satisfied	Somewhat Satisfied	Dissatisfied	Highly Dissatisfied
Entire sample	25.86%	27.59%	34.48%	10.92%	0.57%	0.57%

Table 2.7.2 How satisfied are you that help is there when you need it from the academic library staff? Broken out by country

Country	No Answer	Highly Satisfied	Satisfied	Somewhat Satisfied	Dissatisfied	Highly Dissatisfied
USA	27.27%	28.79%	31.06%	11.36%	0.76%	0.76%
Canada	14.29%	14.29%	57.14%	14.29%	0.00%	0.00%
UK/Ireland	28.00%	16.00%	44.00%	12.00%	0.00%	0.00%
Australia/New Zealand	10.00%	50.00%	40.00%	0.00%	0.00%	0.00%

Table 2.7.3 How satisfied are you that help is there when you need it from the academic library staff? Broken out by US News and World Report World Ranking

US News and World Report World Ranking	No Answer	Highly Satisfied	Satisfied	Somewhat Satisfied	Dissatisfied	Highly Dissatisfied
Less than 25	27.27%	31.82%	29.55%	9.09%	0.00%	2.27%
26 - 90	20.45%	36.36%	29.55%	11.36%	2.27%	0.00%
91 - 135	35.56%	20.00%	37.78%	6.67%	0.00%	0.00%
More than 135	19.51%	21.95%	41.46%	17.07%	0.00%	0.00%

Table 2.7.4 How satisfied are you that help is there when you need it from the academic library staff? Broken out by annual tuition

Annual tuition, $	No Answer	Highly Satisfied	Satisfied	Somewhat Satisfied	Dissatisfied	Highly Dissatisfied
Less than 14500	28.89%	15.56%	42.22%	13.33%	0.00%	0.00%
14500 - 29500	27.91%	23.26%	37.21%	11.63%	0.00%	0.00%
29501 - 45500	20.45%	45.45%	27.27%	4.55%	0.00%	2.27%
More than 45500	26.19%	26.19%	30.95%	14.29%	2.38%	0.00%

Table 2.7.5 How satisfied are you that help is there when you need it from the academic library staff? Broken out by public and private status

Public and private status	No Answer	Highly Satisfied	Satisfied	Somewhat Satisfied	Dissatisfied	Highly Dissatisfied
Public	27.83%	23.48%	36.52%	11.30%	0.00%	0.87%
Private	22.03%	35.59%	30.51%	10.17%	1.69%	0.00%

Table 2.7.6 How satisfied are you that help is there when you need it from the academic library staff? Broken out by gender of the survey participant

You are male or female?	No Answer	Highly Satisfied	Satisfied	Somewhat Satisfied	Dissatisfied	Highly Dissatisfied
Male	29.70%	26.73%	31.68%	10.89%	0.99%	0.00%
Female	20.55%	28.77%	38.36%	10.96%	0.00%	1.37%

Table 2.7.7 How satisfied are you that help is there when you need it from the academic library staff? Broken out by FTE

FTE	No Answer	Highly Satisfied	Satisfied	Somewhat Satisfied	Dissatisfied	Highly Dissatisfied
Less than 8000	28.57%	21.43%	38.10%	11.90%	0.00%	0.00%
8000 - 16000	22.22%	42.22%	28.89%	4.44%	2.22%	0.00%
16001 - 35500	29.55%	18.18%	40.91%	11.36%	0.00%	0.00%
More than 35500	23.26%	27.91%	30.23%	16.28%	0.00%	2.33%

Table 2.7.8 How satisfied are you that help is there when you need it from the academic library staff? Broken out by age range of the survey participant

Which age band best describes you?	No Answer	Highly Satisfied	Satisfied	Somewhat Satisfied	Dissatisfied	Highly Dissatisfied
30 or Under	38.46%	23.08%	38.46%	0.00%	0.00%	0.00%
31 - 39	26.42%	39.62%	20.75%	11.32%	0.00%	1.89%
40 - 49	19.44%	16.67%	47.22%	16.67%	0.00%	0.00%
50 - 59	19.35%	25.81%	38.71%	12.90%	3.23%	0.00%
60 or over	28.57%	25.00%	35.71%	10.71%	0.00%	0.00%

Table 2.7.9 How satisfied are you that help is there when you need it from the academic library staff? Broken out by tenure status

Tenure status	No Answer	Highly Satisfied	Satisfied	Somewhat Satisfied	Dissatisfied	Highly Dissatisfied
Tenured	15.91%	22.73%	52.27%	9.09%	0.00%	0.00%
Not tenured but on a tenure track	33.33%	23.81%	28.57%	14.29%	0.00%	0.00%
Not tenured and not on a tenure track	28.43%	31.37%	27.45%	10.78%	0.98%	0.98%
University does not offer tenure	28.57%	14.29%	42.86%	14.29%	0.00%	0.00%

Table 2.7.10 How satisfied are you that help is there when you need it from the academic library staff? Broken out by academic title of the survey participant

Which phrase best describes your role or title at your university?	No Answer	Highly Satisfied	Satisfied	Somewhat Satisfied	Dissatisfied	Highly Dissatisfied
Professor	25.71%	25.71%	37.14%	11.43%	0.00%	0.00%
Associate Professor or Reader	3.85%	19.23%	65.38%	7.69%	3.85%	0.00%
Assistant Professor	30.95%	23.81%	26.19%	19.05%	0.00%	0.00%
Lecturer or Instructor	33.33%	22.22%	44.44%	0.00%	0.00%	0.00%
Postdoc or Fellow	30.65%	35.48%	24.19%	8.06%	0.00%	1.61%

Table 2.7.11 How satisfied are you that help is there when you need it from the academic library staff? Broken out by school or academic department of the survey participant

Which phrase best describes your academic department?	No Answer	Highly Satisfied	Satisfied	Somewhat Satisfied	Dissatisfied	Highly Dissatisfied
Medical School Department	24.47%	34.04%	27.66%	12.77%	0.00%	1.06%
University Faculty of Biology	38.71%	19.35%	25.81%	16.13%	0.00%	0.00%
University Faculty of Chemistry	46.15%	7.69%	46.15%	0.00%	0.00%	0.00%
Department or School of Public Health, Nursing, Healthcare Informatics	7.41%	22.22%	62.96%	3.70%	3.70%	0.00%
Dentistry	40.00%	40.00%	20.00%	0.00%	0.00%	0.00%
Veterinary	0.00%	25.00%	50.00%	25.00%	0.00%	0.00%

Table 2.8.1 How satisfied are you with the level of physical comfort in the library?

	No Answer	Highly Satisfied	Satisfied	Somewhat Satisfied	Dissatisfied	Highly Dissatisfied
Entire sample	31.61%	20.69%	34.48%	11.49%	1.15%	0.57%

Table 2.8.2 How satisfied are you with the level of physical comfort in the library? Broken out by country

Country	No Answer	Highly Satisfied	Satisfied	Somewhat Satisfied	Dissatisfied	Highly Dissatisfied
USA	32.58%	21.97%	32.58%	11.36%	0.76%	0.76%
Canada	0.00%	28.57%	57.14%	14.29%	0.00%	0.00%
UK/Ireland	40.00%	12.00%	36.00%	12.00%	0.00%	0.00%
Australia/New Zealand	20.00%	20.00%	40.00%	10.00%	10.00%	0.00%

Table 2.8.3 How satisfied are you with the level of physical comfort in the library? Broken out by US News and World Report World Ranking

US News and World Report World Ranking	No Answer	Highly Satisfied	Satisfied	Somewhat Satisfied	Dissatisfied	Highly Dissatisfied
Less than 25	27.27%	29.55%	25.00%	15.91%	0.00%	2.27%
26 - 90	36.36%	22.73%	36.36%	4.55%	0.00%	0.00%
91 - 135	46.67%	13.33%	31.11%	8.89%	0.00%	0.00%
More than 135	14.63%	17.07%	46.34%	17.07%	4.88%	0.00%

Table 2.8.4 How satisfied are you with the level of physical comfort in the library? Broken out by annual tuition

Annual tuition, $	No Answer	Highly Satisfied	Satisfied	Somewhat Satisfied	Dissatisfied	Highly Dissatisfied
Less than 14500	33.33%	13.33%	40.00%	11.11%	2.22%	0.00%
14500 - 29500	32.56%	13.95%	37.21%	16.28%	0.00%	0.00%
29501 - 45500	27.27%	36.36%	25.00%	6.82%	2.27%	2.27%
More than 45500	33.33%	19.05%	35.71%	11.90%	0.00%	0.00%

Table 2.8.5 How satisfied are you with the level of physical comfort in the library? Broken out by public and private status

Public and private status	No Answer	Highly Satisfied	Satisfied	Somewhat Satisfied	Dissatisfied	Highly Dissatisfied
Public	34.78%	16.52%	33.04%	13.04%	1.74%	0.87%
Private	25.42%	28.81%	37.29%	8.47%	0.00%	0.00%

Table 2.8.6 How satisfied are you with the level of physical comfort in the library? Broken out by gender of the survey participant

You are male or female?	No Answer	Highly Satisfied	Satisfied	Somewhat Satisfied	Dissatisfied	Highly Dissatisfied
Male	26.73%	24.75%	34.65%	12.87%	0.99%	0.00%
Female	38.36%	15.07%	34.25%	9.59%	1.37%	1.37%

Table 2.8.7 How satisfied are you with the level of physical comfort in the library? Broken out by FTE

FTE	No Answer	Highly Satisfied	Satisfied	Somewhat Satisfied	Dissatisfied	Highly Dissatisfied
Less than 8000	38.10%	19.05%	30.95%	11.90%	0.00%	0.00%
8000 - 16000	37.78%	28.89%	31.11%	2.22%	0.00%	0.00%
16001 - 35500	22.73%	13.64%	40.91%	18.18%	4.55%	0.00%
More than 35500	27.91%	20.93%	34.88%	13.95%	0.00%	2.33%

Table 2.8.8 How satisfied are you with the level of physical comfort in the library? Broken out by age range of the survey participant

Which age band best describes you?	No Answer	Highly Satisfied	Satisfied	Somewhat Satisfied	Dissatisfied	Highly Dissatisfied
30 or Under	46.15%	15.38%	38.46%	0.00%	0.00%	0.00%
31 - 39	37.74%	24.53%	20.75%	15.09%	0.00%	1.89%
40 - 49	27.78%	19.44%	38.89%	13.89%	0.00%	0.00%
50 - 59	12.90%	12.90%	54.84%	12.90%	6.45%	0.00%
60 or over	32.14%	28.57%	28.57%	10.71%	0.00%	0.00%

Table 2.8.9 How satisfied are you with the level of physical comfort in the library? Broken out by tenure status

Tenure status	No Answer	Highly Satisfied	Satisfied	Somewhat Satisfied	Dissatisfied	Highly Dissatisfied
Tenured	15.91%	15.91%	52.27%	11.36%	4.55%	0.00%
Not tenured but on a tenure track	38.10%	19.05%	28.57%	14.29%	0.00%	0.00%
Not tenured and not on a tenure track	37.25%	23.53%	30.39%	7.84%	0.00%	0.98%
University does not offer tenure	28.57%	14.29%	0.00%	57.14%	0.00%	0.00%

Table 2.8.10 How satisfied are you with the level of physical comfort in the library? Broken out by academic title of the survey participant

Which phrase best describes your role or title at your university?	No Answer	Highly Satisfied	Satisfied	Somewhat Satisfied	Dissatisfied	Highly Dissatisfied
Professor	20.00%	28.57%	37.14%	11.43%	2.86%	0.00%
Associate Professor or Reader	11.54%	11.54%	61.54%	11.54%	3.85%	0.00%
Assistant Professor	42.86%	11.90%	23.81%	21.43%	0.00%	0.00%
Lecturer or Instructor	22.22%	11.11%	66.67%	0.00%	0.00%	0.00%
Postdoc or Fellow	40.32%	27.42%	24.19%	6.45%	0.00%	1.61%

Table 2.8.11 How satisfied are you with the level of physical comfort in the library? Broken out by school or academic department of the survey participant

Which phrase best describes your academic department?	No Answer	Highly Satisfied	Satisfied	Somewhat Satisfied	Dissatisfied	Highly Dissatisfied
Medical School Department	31.91%	26.60%	26.60%	12.77%	1.06%	1.06%
University Faculty of Biology	48.39%	12.90%	35.48%	3.23%	0.00%	0.00%
University Faculty of Chemistry	38.46%	15.38%	30.77%	15.38%	0.00%	0.00%
Department or School of Public Health, Nursing, Healthcare Informatics	14.81%	7.41%	62.96%	11.11%	3.70%	0.00%
Dentistry	20.00%	40.00%	20.00%	20.00%	0.00%	0.00%
Veterinary	0.00%	25.00%	50.00%	25.00%	0.00%	0.00%

Table 2.9.1 How satisfied are you with your academic library's capabilities in training students in research skills?

	No Answer	Highly Satisfied	Satisfied	Somewhat Satisfied	Dissatisfied	Highly Dissatisfied
Entire sample	41.38%	13.22%	29.89%	12.07%	2.87%	0.57%

Table 2.9.2 How satisfied are you with your academic library's capabilities in training students in research skills? Broken out by country

Country	No Answer	Highly Satisfied	Satisfied	Somewhat Satisfied	Dissatisfied	Highly Dissatisfied
USA	46.21%	12.88%	25.00%	12.12%	3.03%	0.76%
Canada	14.29%	28.57%	42.86%	14.29%	0.00%	0.00%
UK/Ireland	32.00%	8.00%	40.00%	16.00%	4.00%	0.00%
Australia/New Zealand	20.00%	20.00%	60.00%	0.00%	0.00%	0.00%

Table 2.9.3 How satisfied are you with your academic library's capabilities in training students in research skills? Broken out by US News and World Report World Ranking

US News and World Report World Ranking	No Answer	Highly Satisfied	Satisfied	Somewhat Satisfied	Dissatisfied	Highly Dissatisfied
Less than 25	40.91%	18.18%	20.45%	18.18%	0.00%	2.27%
26 - 90	47.73%	15.91%	25.00%	9.09%	2.27%	0.00%
91 - 135	48.89%	4.44%	35.56%	6.67%	4.44%	0.00%
More than 135	26.83%	14.63%	39.02%	14.63%	4.88%	0.00%

Table 2.9.4 How satisfied are you with your academic library's capabilities in training students in research skills? Broken out by annual tuition

Annual tuition, $	No Answer	Highly Satisfied	Satisfied	Somewhat Satisfied	Dissatisfied	Highly Dissatisfied
Less than 14500	33.33%	8.89%	42.22%	11.11%	4.44%	0.00%
14500 - 29500	44.19%	9.30%	25.58%	13.95%	6.98%	0.00%
29501 - 45500	40.91%	27.27%	25.00%	4.55%	0.00%	2.27%
More than 45500	47.62%	7.14%	26.19%	19.05%	0.00%	0.00%

Table 2.9.5 How satisfied are you with your academic library's capabilities in training students in research skills? Broken out by public and private status

Public and private status	No Answer	Highly Satisfied	Satisfied	Somewhat Satisfied	Dissatisfied	Highly Dissatisfied
Public	40.00%	13.04%	29.57%	12.17%	4.35%	0.87%
Private	44.07%	13.56%	30.51%	11.86%	0.00%	0.00%

Table 2.9.6 How satisfied are you with your academic library's capabilities in training students in research skills? Broken out by gender of the survey participant

You are male or female?	No Answer	Highly Satisfied	Satisfied	Somewhat Satisfied	Dissatisfied	Highly Dissatisfied
Male	39.60%	13.86%	31.68%	11.88%	2.97%	0.00%
Female	43.84%	12.33%	27.40%	12.33%	2.74%	1.37%

Table 2.9.7 How satisfied are you with your academic library's capabilities in training students in research skills? Broken out by FTE

FTE	No Answer	Highly Satisfied	Satisfied	Somewhat Satisfied	Dissatisfied	Highly Dissatisfied
Less than 8000	38.10%	9.52%	38.10%	7.14%	7.14%	0.00%
8000 - 16000	53.33%	15.56%	22.22%	8.89%	0.00%	0.00%
16001 - 35500	31.82%	13.64%	36.36%	18.18%	0.00%	0.00%
More than 35500	41.86%	13.95%	23.26%	13.95%	4.65%	2.33%

Table 2.9.8 How satisfied are you with your academic library's capabilities in training students in research skills? Broken out by age range of the survey participant

Which age band best describes you?	No Answer	Highly Satisfied	Satisfied	Somewhat Satisfied	Dissatisfied	Highly Dissatisfied
30 or Under	42.31%	15.38%	34.62%	7.69%	0.00%	0.00%
31 - 39	45.28%	18.87%	20.75%	11.32%	1.89%	1.89%
40 - 49	44.44%	5.56%	25.00%	19.44%	5.56%	0.00%
50 - 59	29.03%	9.68%	51.61%	6.45%	3.23%	0.00%
60 or over	42.86%	14.29%	25.00%	14.29%	3.57%	0.00%

Table 2.9.9 How satisfied are you with your academic library's capabilities in training students in research skills? Broken out by tenure status

Tenure status	No Answer	Highly Satisfied	Satisfied	Somewhat Satisfied	Dissatisfied	Highly Dissatisfied
Tenured	27.27%	11.36%	40.91%	18.18%	2.27%	0.00%
Not tenured but on a tenure track	57.14%	9.52%	14.29%	14.29%	4.76%	0.00%
Not tenured and not on a tenure track	44.12%	15.69%	26.47%	9.80%	2.94%	0.98%
University does not offer tenure	42.86%	0.00%	57.14%	0.00%	0.00%	0.00%

Table 2.9.10 How satisfied are you with your academic library's capabilities in training students in research skills? Broken out by academic title of the survey participant

Which phrase best describes your role or title at your university?	No Answer	Highly Satisfied	Satisfied	Somewhat Satisfied	Dissatisfied	Highly Dissatisfied
Professor	37.14%	11.43%	34.29%	17.14%	0.00%	0.00%
Associate Professor or Reader	34.62%	3.85%	46.15%	11.54%	3.85%	0.00%
Assistant Professor	52.38%	7.14%	19.05%	11.90%	9.52%	0.00%
Lecturer or Instructor	22.22%	11.11%	66.67%	0.00%	0.00%	0.00%
Postdoc or Fellow	41.94%	22.58%	22.58%	11.29%	0.00%	1.61%

Table 2.9.11 How satisfied are you with your academic library's capabilities in training students in research skills? Broken out by school or academic department of the survey participant

Which phrase best describes your academic department?	No Answer	Highly Satisfied	Satisfied	Somewhat Satisfied	Dissatisfied	Highly Dissatisfied
Medical School Department	45.74%	15.96%	22.34%	10.64%	4.26%	1.06%
University Faculty of Biology	48.39%	6.45%	32.26%	9.68%	3.23%	0.00%
University Faculty of Chemistry	46.15%	7.69%	30.77%	15.38%	0.00%	0.00%
Department or School of Public Health, Nursing, Healthcare Informatics	18.52%	7.41%	62.96%	11.11%	0.00%	0.00%
Dentistry	40.00%	40.00%	0.00%	20.00%	0.00%	0.00%
Veterinary	25.00%	25.00%	0.00%	50.00%	0.00%	0.00%

Table 2.10.1 How satisfied are you with your academic library's general reference services?

	No Answer	Highly Satisfied	Satisfied	Somewhat Satisfied	Dissatisfied	Highly Dissatisfied
Entire sample	29.31%	20.69%	38.51%	9.20%	1.72%	0.57%

Table 2.10.2 How satisfied are you with your academic library's general reference services? Broken out by country

Country	No Answer	Highly Satisfied	Satisfied	Somewhat Satisfied	Dissatisfied	Highly Dissatisfied
USA	31.06%	22.73%	33.33%	9.85%	2.27%	0.76%
Canada	28.57%	14.29%	42.86%	14.29%	0.00%	0.00%
UK/Ireland	32.00%	12.00%	48.00%	8.00%	0.00%	0.00%
Australia/New Zealand	0.00%	20.00%	80.00%	0.00%	0.00%	0.00%

Table 2.10.3 How satisfied are you with your academic library's general reference services? Broken out by US News and World Report World Ranking

US News and World Report World Ranking	No Answer	Highly Satisfied	Satisfied	Somewhat Satisfied	Dissatisfied	Highly Dissatisfied
Less than 25	27.27%	27.27%	29.55%	13.64%	0.00%	2.27%
26 - 90	29.55%	29.55%	34.09%	4.55%	2.27%	0.00%
91 - 135	37.78%	15.56%	35.56%	6.67%	4.44%	0.00%
More than 135	21.95%	9.76%	56.10%	12.20%	0.00%	0.00%

Table 2.10.4 How satisfied are you with your academic library's general reference services? Broken out by annual tuition

Annual tuition, $	No Answer	Highly Satisfied	Satisfied	Somewhat Satisfied	Dissatisfied	Highly Dissatisfied
Less than 14500	33.33%	11.11%	46.67%	6.67%	2.22%	0.00%
14500 - 29500	30.23%	16.28%	39.53%	11.63%	2.33%	0.00%
29501 - 45500	20.45%	38.64%	34.09%	4.55%	0.00%	2.27%
More than 45500	33.33%	16.67%	33.33%	14.29%	2.38%	0.00%

Table 2.10.5 How satisfied are you with your academic library's general reference services? Broken out by public and private status

Public and private status	No Answer	Highly Satisfied	Satisfied	Somewhat Satisfied	Dissatisfied	Highly Dissatisfied
Public	30.43%	18.26%	39.13%	9.57%	1.74%	0.87%
Private	27.12%	25.42%	37.29%	8.47%	1.69%	0.00%

Table 2.10.6 How satisfied are you with your academic library's general reference services? Broken out by gender of the survey participant

You are male or female?	No Answer	Highly Satisfied	Satisfied	Somewhat Satisfied	Dissatisfied	Highly Dissatisfied
Male	28.71%	23.76%	34.65%	10.89%	1.98%	0.00%
Female	30.14%	16.44%	43.84%	6.85%	1.37%	1.37%

Table 2.10.7 How satisfied are you with your academic library's general reference services? Broken out by FTE

FTE	No Answer	Highly Satisfied	Satisfied	Somewhat Satisfied	Dissatisfied	Highly Dissatisfied
Less than 8000	28.57%	19.05%	38.10%	9.52%	4.76%	0.00%
8000 - 16000	33.33%	28.89%	33.33%	2.22%	2.22%	0.00%
16001 - 35500	27.27%	15.91%	43.18%	13.64%	0.00%	0.00%
More than 35500	27.91%	18.60%	39.53%	11.63%	0.00%	2.33%

Table 2.10.8 How satisfied are you with your academic library's general reference services? Broken out by age range of the survey participant

Which age band best describes you?	No Answer	Highly Satisfied	Satisfied	Somewhat Satisfied	Dissatisfied	Highly Dissatisfied
30 or Under	46.15%	19.23%	26.92%	7.69%	0.00%	0.00%
31 - 39	26.42%	33.96%	26.42%	9.43%	1.89%	1.89%
40 - 49	27.78%	11.11%	50.00%	11.11%	0.00%	0.00%
50 - 59	19.35%	9.68%	61.29%	6.45%	3.23%	0.00%
60 or over	32.14%	21.43%	32.14%	10.71%	3.57%	0.00%

Table 2.10.9 How satisfied are you with your academic library's general reference services? Broken out by Tenure status

Tenure status	No Answer	Highly Satisfied	Satisfied	Somewhat Satisfied	Dissatisfied	Highly Dissatisfied
Tenured	18.18%	13.64%	56.82%	11.36%	0.00%	0.00%
Not tenured but on a tenure track	28.57%	19.05%	42.86%	9.52%	0.00%	0.00%
Not tenured and not on a tenure track	34.31%	24.51%	29.41%	7.84%	2.94%	0.98%
University does not offer tenure	28.57%	14.29%	42.86%	14.29%	0.00%	0.00%

Table 2.10.10 How satisfied are you with your academic library's general reference services? Broken out by academic title of the survey participant

Which phrase best describes your role or title at your university?	No Answer	Highly Satisfied	Satisfied	Somewhat Satisfied	Dissatisfied	Highly Dissatisfied
Professor	25.71%	17.14%	48.57%	8.57%	0.00%	0.00%
Associate Professor or Reader	11.54%	11.54%	61.54%	7.69%	7.69%	0.00%
Assistant Professor	33.33%	16.67%	33.33%	14.29%	2.38%	0.00%
Lecturer or Instructor	22.22%	22.22%	55.56%	0.00%	0.00%	0.00%
Postdoc or Fellow	37.10%	29.03%	24.19%	8.06%	0.00%	1.61%

Table 2.10.11 How satisfied are you with your academic library's general reference services? Broken out by school or academic department of the survey participant

Which phrase best describes your academic department?	No Answer	Highly Satisfied	Satisfied	Somewhat Satisfied	Dissatisfied	Highly Dissatisfied
Medical School Department	32.98%	24.47%	28.72%	11.70%	1.06%	1.06%
University Faculty of Biology	45.16%	16.13%	35.48%	3.23%	0.00%	0.00%
University Faculty of Chemistry	23.08%	15.38%	46.15%	15.38%	0.00%	0.00%
Department or School of Public Health, Nursing, Healthcare Informatics	7.41%	11.11%	74.07%	0.00%	7.41%	0.00%
Dentistry	20.00%	40.00%	20.00%	20.00%	0.00%	0.00%
Veterinary	0.00%	25.00%	50.00%	25.00%	0.00%	0.00%

Table 2.11.1 How satisfied are you with the quality and range of information technology made available to you in the library?

	No Answer	Highly Satisfied	Satisfied	Somewhat Satisfied	Dissatisfied	Highly Dissatisfied
Entire sample	28.16%	21.84%	37.93%	10.92%	0.00%	1.15%

Table 2.11.2 How satisfied are you with the quality and range of information technology made available to you in the library? Broken out by country

Country	No Answer	Highly Satisfied	Satisfied	Somewhat Satisfied	Dissatisfied	Highly Dissatisfied
USA	29.55%	23.48%	35.61%	9.85%	0.00%	1.52%
Canada	28.57%	28.57%	28.57%	14.29%	0.00%	0.00%
UK/Ireland	28.00%	16.00%	40.00%	16.00%	0.00%	0.00%
Australia/New Zealand	10.00%	10.00%	70.00%	10.00%	0.00%	0.00%

Table 2.11.3 How satisfied are you with the quality and range of information technology made available to you in the library? Broken out by US News and World Report World Ranking

US News and World Report World Ranking	No Answer	Highly Satisfied	Satisfied	Somewhat Satisfied	Dissatisfied	Highly Dissatisfied
Less than 25	25.00%	27.27%	34.09%	11.36%	0.00%	2.27%
26 - 90	22.73%	29.55%	38.64%	6.82%	0.00%	2.27%
91 - 135	40.00%	17.78%	31.11%	11.11%	0.00%	0.00%
More than 135	24.39%	12.20%	48.78%	14.63%	0.00%	0.00%

Table 2.11.4 How satisfied are you with the quality and range of information technology made available to you in the library? Broken out by annual tuition

Annual tuition, $	No Answer	Highly Satisfied	Satisfied	Somewhat Satisfied	Dissatisfied	Highly Dissatisfied
Less than 14500	33.33%	13.33%	40.00%	13.33%	0.00%	0.00%
14500 - 29500	34.88%	16.28%	41.86%	6.98%	0.00%	0.00%
29501 - 45500	20.45%	36.36%	27.27%	13.64%	0.00%	2.27%
More than 45500	23.81%	21.43%	42.86%	9.52%	0.00%	2.38%

Table 2.11.5 How satisfied are you with the quality and range of information technology made available to you in the library? Broken out by public and private status

Public and private status	No Answer	Highly Satisfied	Satisfied	Somewhat Satisfied	Dissatisfied	Highly Dissatisfied
Public	32.17%	18.26%	37.39%	11.30%	0.00%	0.87%
Private	20.34%	28.81%	38.98%	10.17%	0.00%	1.69%

Table 2.11.6 How satisfied are you with the quality and range of information technology made available to you in the library? Broken out by gender of the survey participant

You are male or female?	No Answer	Highly Satisfied	Satisfied	Somewhat Satisfied	Dissatisfied	Highly Dissatisfied
Male	27.72%	25.74%	35.64%	9.90%	0.00%	0.99%
Female	28.77%	16.44%	41.10%	12.33%	0.00%	1.37%

Table 2.11.7 How satisfied are you with the quality and range of information technology made available to you in the library? Broken out by FTE

FTE	No Answer	Highly Satisfied	Satisfied	Somewhat Satisfied	Dissatisfied	Highly Dissatisfied
Less than 8000	33.33%	21.43%	33.33%	11.90%	0.00%	0.00%
8000 - 16000	22.22%	31.11%	37.78%	6.67%	0.00%	2.22%
16001 - 35500	31.82%	11.36%	43.18%	13.64%	0.00%	0.00%
More than 35500	25.58%	23.26%	37.21%	11.63%	0.00%	2.33%

Table 2.11.8 How satisfied are you with the quality and range of information technology made available to you in the library? Broken out by age range of the survey participant

Which age band best describes you:	No Answer	Highly Satisfied	Satisfied	Somewhat Satisfied	Dissatisfied	Highly Dissatisfied
30 or Under	42.31%	23.08%	30.77%	3.85%	0.00%	0.00%
31 - 39	28.30%	32.08%	32.08%	5.66%	0.00%	1.89%
40 - 49	22.22%	13.89%	41.67%	22.22%	0.00%	0.00%
50 - 59	22.58%	16.13%	41.94%	16.13%	0.00%	3.23%
60 or over	28.57%	17.86%	46.43%	7.14%	0.00%	0.00%

Table 2.11.9 How satisfied are you with the quality and range of information technology made available to you in the library? Broken out by tenure status

Tenure status	No Answer	Highly Satisfied	Satisfied	Somewhat Satisfied	Dissatisfied	Highly Dissatisfied
Tenured	20.45%	13.64%	50.00%	15.91%	0.00%	0.00%
Not tenured but on a tenure track	28.57%	23.81%	38.10%	9.52%	0.00%	0.00%
Not tenured and not on a tenure track	31.37%	26.47%	32.35%	7.84%	0.00%	1.96%
University does not offer tenure	28.57%	0.00%	42.86%	28.57%	0.00%	0.00%

Table 2.11.10 How satisfied are you with the quality and range of information technology made available to you in the library? Broken out by academic title of the survey participant

Which phrase best describes your role or title at your university?	No Answer	Highly Satisfied	Satisfied	Somewhat Satisfied	Dissatisfied	Highly Dissatisfied
Professor	28.57%	25.71%	40.00%	5.71%	0.00%	0.00%
Associate Professor or Reader	7.69%	7.69%	53.85%	26.92%	0.00%	3.85%
Assistant Professor	33.33%	14.29%	40.48%	11.90%	0.00%	0.00%
Lecturer or Instructor	22.22%	22.22%	55.56%	0.00%	0.00%	0.00%
Postdoc or Fellow	33.87%	30.65%	25.81%	8.06%	0.00%	1.61%

Table 2.11.11 How satisfied are you with the quality and range of information technology made available to you in the library? Broken out by school or academic department of the survey participant

Which phrase best describes your academic department?	No Answer	Highly Satisfied	Satisfied	Somewhat Satisfied	Dissatisfied	Highly Dissatisfied
Medical School Department	30.85%	25.53%	30.85%	11.70%	0.00%	1.06%
University Faculty of Biology	38.71%	19.35%	32.26%	9.68%	0.00%	0.00%
University Faculty of Chemistry	30.77%	15.38%	46.15%	7.69%	0.00%	0.00%
Department or School of Public Health, Nursing, Healthcare Informatics	11.11%	11.11%	70.37%	3.70%	0.00%	3.70%
Dentistry	20.00%	40.00%	20.00%	20.00%	0.00%	0.00%
Veterinary	0.00%	25.00%	25.00%	50.00%	0.00%	0.00%

Table 3.1 Compared to other services and departments connected to the life sciences faculty at your university the library is generally more efficient, as efficient or less efficient?

	No Answer	Less Efficient	As Efficient	More Efficient
Entire sample	13.22%	4.02%	59.77%	22.99%

Table 3.2 Compared to other services and departments connected to the life sciences faculty at your university the library is generally more efficient, as efficient or less efficient? Broken out by country

Country	No Answer	Less Efficient	As Efficient	More Efficient
USA	15.15%	4.55%	56.06%	24.24%
Canada	0.00%	0.00%	71.43%	28.57%
UK/Ireland	12.00%	4.00%	68.00%	16.00%
Australia/New Zealand	0.00%	0.00%	80.00%	20.00%

Table 3.3 Compared to other services and departments connected to the life sciences faculty at your university the library is generally more efficient, as efficient or less efficient? Broken out by US News and World Report World Ranking

US News and World Report World Ranking	No Answer	Less Efficient	As Efficient	More Efficient
Less than 25	18.18%	2.27%	54.55%	25.00%
26 - 90	4.55%	6.82%	61.36%	27.27%
91 - 135	28.89%	4.44%	51.11%	15.56%
More than 135	0.00%	2.44%	73.17%	24.39%

Table 3.4 Compared to other services and departments connected to the life sciences faculty at your university the library is generally more efficient, as efficient or less efficient? Broken out by Annual tuition, $

Annual tuition, $	No Answer	Less Efficient	As Efficient	More Efficient
Less than 14500	13.33%	2.22%	64.44%	20.00%
14500 - 29500	20.93%	11.63%	53.49%	13.95%
29501 - 45500	4.55%	2.27%	61.36%	31.82%
More than 45500	14.29%	0.00%	59.52%	26.19%

Table 3.5 Compared to other services and departments connected to the life sciences faculty at your university the library is generally more efficient, as efficient or less efficient? Broken out by public and private status

Public and private status	No Answer	Less Efficient	As Efficient	More Efficient
Public	13.91%	5.22%	61.74%	19.13%
Private	11.86%	1.69%	55.93%	30.51%

Table 3.6 Compared to other services and departments connected to the life sciences faculty at your university the library is generally more efficient, as efficient or less efficient? Broken out by gender of the survey participant

You are male or female?	No Answer	Less Efficient	As Efficient	More Efficient
Male	13.86%	3.96%	59.41%	22.77%
Female	12.33%	4.11%	60.27%	23.29%

Table 3.7 Compared to other services and departments connected to the life sciences faculty at your university the library is generally more efficient, as efficient or less efficient? Broken out by FTE

FTE	No Answer	Less Efficient	As Efficient	More Efficient
Less than 8000	21.43%	7.14%	42.86%	28.57%
8000 - 16000	11.11%	4.44%	55.56%	28.89%
16001 - 35500	6.82%	2.27%	81.82%	9.09%
More than 35500	13.95%	2.33%	58.14%	25.58%

Table 3.8 Compared to other services and departments connected to the life sciences faculty at your university the library is generally Broken out by age range of the survey participant

Which age band best describes you:	No Answer	Less Efficient	As Efficient	More Efficient
30 or Under	19.23%	7.69%	53.85%	19.23%
31 - 39	13.21%	3.77%	60.38%	22.64%
40 - 49	8.33%	8.33%	63.89%	19.44%
50 - 59	6.45%	0.00%	58.06%	35.48%
60 or over	21.43%	0.00%	60.71%	17.86%

Table 3.9 Compared to other services and departments connected to the life sciences faculty at your university the library is generally more efficient, as efficient or less efficient? Broken out by tenure status

Tenure status	No Answer	Less Efficient	As Efficient	More Efficient
Tenured	4.55%	2.27%	68.18%	25.00%
Not tenured but on a tenure track	4.76%	9.52%	71.43%	14.29%
Not tenured and not on a tenure track	18.63%	3.92%	53.92%	23.53%
University does not offer tenure	14.29%	0.00%	57.14%	28.57%

Table 3.10 Compared to other services and departments connected to the life sciences faculty at your university the library is generally more efficient, as efficient or less efficient? Broken out by academic title of the survey participant

Which phrase best describes your role or title at your university?	No Answer	Less Efficient	As Efficient	More Efficient
Professor	11.43%	2.86%	60.00%	25.71%
Associate Professor or Reader	3.85%	0.00%	73.08%	23.08%
Assistant Professor	11.90%	9.52%	64.29%	14.29%
Lecturer or Instructor	11.11%	0.00%	77.78%	11.11%
Postdoc or Fellow	19.35%	3.23%	48.39%	29.03%

Table 3.11 Compared to other services and departments connected to the life sciences faculty at your university the library is generally more efficient, as efficient or less efficient? Broken out by school or academic department of the survey participant

Which phrase best describes your academic department?	No Answer	Less Efficient	As Efficient	More Efficient
Medical School Department	14.89%	4.26%	53.19%	27.66%
University Faculty of Biology	19.35%	3.23%	67.74%	9.68%
University Faculty of Chemistry	15.38%	7.69%	61.54%	15.38%
Department or School of Public Health, Nursing, Healthcare Informatics	0.00%	3.70%	70.37%	25.93%
Dentistry	20.00%	0.00%	40.00%	40.00%
Veterinary	0.00%	0.00%	100.00%	0.00%

Made in United States
North Haven, CT
04 November 2026

21727480R00052